Yoga: Yoga for Beginners: The Essential Poses for All Beginners, with Pictures

Yoga for Weight Loss, Anxiety and Stress Relief

Table of contents

Introduction

Chapter 1: Yoga Is More Than Just Poses

Chapter 2: What Is Yoga?

Chapter 3: Yoga and Health Benefits

Chapter 4: Flexibility

Chapter 5: Weight loss

Chapter 6: Relaxed State of Mind

Chapter 7: Emotional Stability

Chapter 8: Improved Posture

Chapter 9: Why Do Yoga?

Chapter 10: Top 20 Yoga Poses for Beginners

Conclusion and Thank You!

My Other Best Selling Books!

Introduction

I want to thank and congratulate you for purchasing the book, "Yoga: Yoga for Beginners: The Essential Poses for All Beginners, with Pictures".

This book contains proven steps and strategies on how to perform the essential yoga poses that every beginner should know. These poses help with weight loss, releasing stress and anxiety, and overall improving your health. We picked the best poses that are simple, and offer the greatest benefit without intimidating the beginner. We also included a lot of useful information on yoga so you can have a better understanding of all the benefits. I truly feel this book is useful for any beginner, and is even a great refresher for the more advanced!

Thanks again for purchasing this book, I hope this book helps you!

Chapter 1: Yoga Is More Than Just Poses

Have you ever wished you had that one golden formula to help advance your mind, body and spirit? What would you first do if that formula was right in front of you? Would you do everything you can to reach your goals? Or would you find an excuse, consider it as too good to be true and simply pass it off? Yoga allows you to reach your fitness goals right at home! Not only can it help build your strength, but flexibility and posture as well. Equally as important, yoga helps reduces stress and anxiety. The benefits of doing yoga are endless.

Yoga is much more than just poses. When you hear the word yoga, the first thing that comes to mind might be a bunch of poses. Yoga is much more than just poses! Yoga is an ancient technique considered as a method of discipline. This technique is not only focused on increasing ones flexibility and inner strength, it also revolves around the purpose of giving you a profound change in your life. Yoga is a transformation that touches all aspects of your life. There is a reason this technique is also deemed as the ultimate spiritual discipline.

Chapter 2: What Is Yoga?

Yoga has been in existence for thousands of years. In fact, there were artifacts found back in 3000 B.C. demonstrating yoga poses. This is a practice passed on from one experienced teacher to devoted students. Yoga has a lot of interpretation; some considers it as a method of discipline and unity. Others believe it to be the most effective technique in terms of strength, meditation, relaxation and more. In this modern day, yoga is perceived as one of the most enduring types of exercises.

Yoga has massive beneficial effects on the mind and body, and there are more than one hundred types of yoga. The form of yoga to choose will depend on your goals. If you want to focus more on your muscles, and burn a large amount of calories, you might want to try the power form of yoga. If you want to achieve a peaceful mind, and master some breathing techniques, you can try ashtanga yoga. If you want to start with basic movements and breathing techniques, hatha is a good choice. As you can see, there are many yoga forms to discover and try, so you are assured that yoga can offer a many benefits.

Chapter 3: Yoga and Health Benefits

If you are a beginner yoga practitioner, you might be skeptical of all the benefits. Don't give up yet! Yoga requires concentration, and once you fully commit yourself to this form of exercise, you might never want to go back to your old exercise routine. Here are some of the health benefits of yoga.

Chapter 4: Flexibility

Yoga undeniably plays a vital role in achieving an impressive stretch you never thought was possible. In stretching, there are three important connective tissues you need to familiarize yourself with. These include you tendons, your ligaments and your muscle fascia.

Your tendons are responsible for connecting your muscles to your bones. They are made of really strong connective tissues, which are built to withstand certain amounts of tension. However, if you understand how your body works you will come to realize that tendons can only be stretched to certain level. Stretching your tendons more than its capacity of 4% might lead to tear.

Ligaments are another form of connective tissue that are more flexible than your tendons. Science will tell you that your ligaments are responsible for holding together your bones, cartilages and joints. They have more stretching capacity then your tendons but still have limitations when it comes to stretching percentage.

Muscle fascia is a group of connective tissue that separates your muscles from your organs internally. It comes in three different types, the superficial, deep and visceral fascia. This group of tissue plays a major role when it comes to flexibility.

The truth is, you were born with the ability to stretch! In your mother's womb you flexed so much that you fit comfortably inside the uterus! Imagine the fetal position where most of your muscles were stretched comfortably. Unfortunately, after several years outside the womb you eventually lose that ability. With yoga practice, achieving that impressive flexibility once again is possible.

You see, yoga helps you better connect with your body, therefore realizing that you're about to trigger an injury in advance. This is what yoga can do to avoid tendon, ligament and muscle fascia damage. Meditation, breathing techniques and a state of calm body and mind can help you stretch without causing any damage to your connective tissues. This is how yoga enhances your flexibility.

Chapter 5: Weight loss

Yoga can definitely be used as a form of weight loss. It helps reduce weight not by incorporating vigorous physical exercises, which is the traditional way of losing weight. With yoga, your presence of mind is more awake, leading to a more conscious effort when it comes to eating habits and choices. Yoga also reduces amount of stress through relaxation techniques, and as a result you seek to eat healthier which reduces weight, rather than stress eating.

According to the American College of Sports Medicine, yoga promotes aerobic exercise that is responsible for effective weight loss. Aerobic exercise requires the use of large muscle groups; it has great impact on your heart and lungs. To lose weight and burn calories effectively, you need to ensure your heart works hard and beats faster.

With yoga you can work your heart as if you're doing extreme physical exercises through the use of power yoga. This form of yoga focuses more on exercise with high intensity and is quite fast paced. Note that yoga has more than one hundred forms. Some are better for beginners, while others are better for the advanced.

Chapter 6: Relaxed State of Mind

You have experienced anxiety at some point in your life. You have probably also felt high stress as well. These are all parts of living, and this is why you need yoga to attain the highest form of relaxation you need. Yoga helps you attain a state of calmness, which at the same time provides you the needed strength to face your daily battles. Yoga enhances your ability to let go of worrisome thoughts. Breathing techniques are also useful. Breathing and yoga go hand in hand.

Chapter 7: Emotional Stability

Yoga, meditation and mindful practice help achieve the emotional stability you need. It has strong effects on your body where it can regulate your emotions and energies effectively. Research shows that too much emotional stress can possibly affect vital organs in your body. Yoga can help manage your emotions, which then lead to emotional stability, and later on to optimal functions of your internal organs. There are specific yoga poses that can really stabilize your emotional level and regulate energy-centered organs such as your spleen, kidneys and lungs.

Chapter 8: Improved Posture

Have you noticed that celebrities practicing yoga have impressive body postures despite their age? Although age is one major factor that can affect your health, there are a few ways to delay the aging effects. Yes, yoga can improve your posture. There are many exercises that counteract your body's tendency for bad postures, like slouching. Yoga increases body awareness, which is a big factor in improving your posture.

Chapter 9: Why Do Yoga?

Yoga has a lot of health benefits, and this is why you should do it. It helps you address so many issues in your life, not only the physical aspect, but also mental, spiritual and emotional aspects. Take your time to perform yoga poses and stretches. Little by little you are improving your life without being too hard on yourself. So let's explore the different basic yoga poses, and achieve a balanced state of body and mind.

Chapter 10: Top 20 Yoga Poses for Beginners

Settle down, don't get too excited! Before trying out some of the top basic yoga poses on your own, you might want to assess your body's ability. See what yoga postures you think you are capable of. Avoid poses and stretches that you think you can't handle just yet. Remember not to force your body to try on some yoga forms that may lead to injuries rather than benefits.

If you are a beginner, here are some of the best yoga poses you can try. Never rush when trying out yoga, and remember to observe the right balance and breathing with these basic and common postures. Hold each pose for as long as you feel comfortable.

1.   Child's Pose

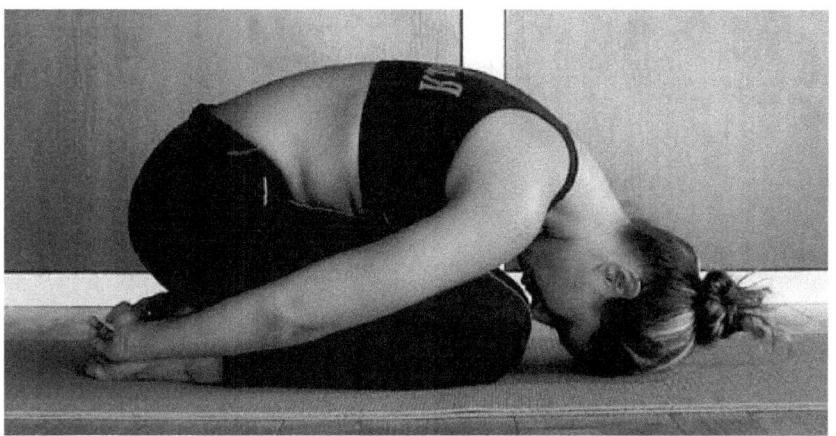

Photo Source: Wikimedia Commons

This pose is rated as one of the easiest and basic yoga poses. Its Sanskrit name is "Bala-asana" which means child.

Instructions:

- Sit on both knees with your buttocks on your heels comfortably resting. Ensure your knees are separated the same as your hip width. Rest your hands with palms facing down on your thighs.

- Inhale slowly and deeply. Make sure to exhale as you slowly bring your chest forward right between your knees, and at the same time bringing your arms forward.

- As soon as your forehead reaches the floor, rest and bring your arms to the sides of your feet with palms facing up. Hold your posture for at least one or two minutes and return to your kneeling position.

2.   The Lotus Pose

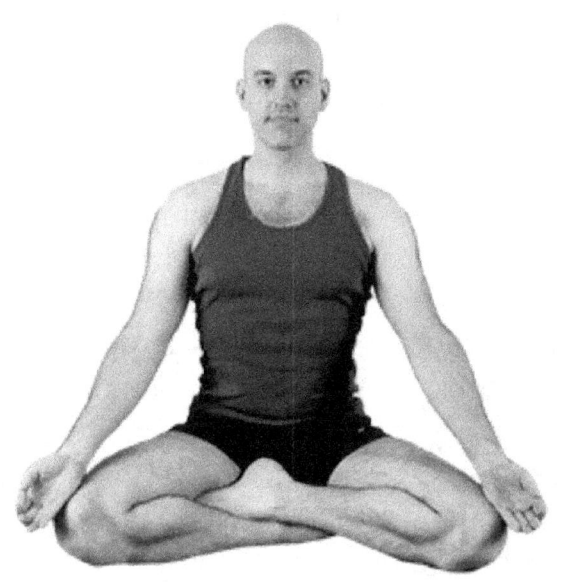

Photo Source: Wikimedia Commons

This pose looks simple; it can be done depending on the flexibility of your legs. You may need to build up flexibility first. Its Sanskrit name is "Padma-asana." Doing this pose resembles a beautiful lotus flower.

Instructions:

- Sit with spine properly straight and comfortably cross your legs.

- Make sure your left foot is perfectly resting right above your right thigh and vice versa. As much as possible, bring your left and right foot closer to your navel and your soles must be pointed in upward direction. This pose is usually used to meditate.

- Your hands must be resting on your knees with your palms facing upward. Don't forget to form a small circle using your thumb and forefinger while extending the rest of your fingers. You can freely switch your leg position if you feel uncomfortable.

3. The Wind Releasing Pose

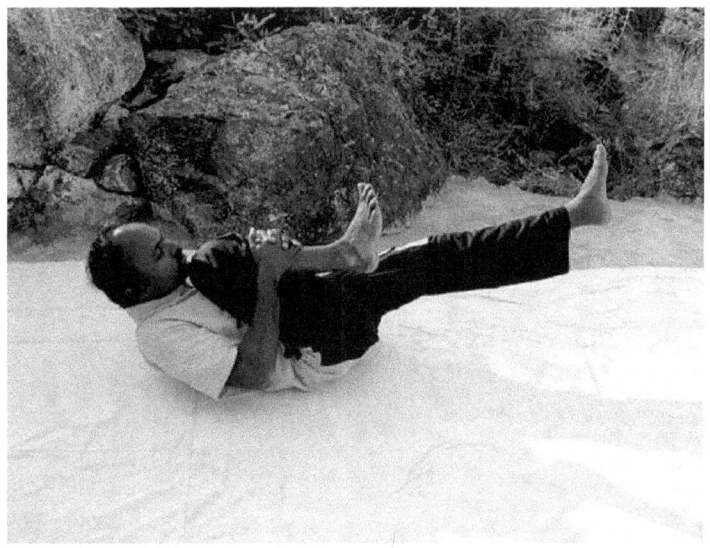

Photo Source: Wikimedia Commons

From its Sanskrit name "Pavana-mukta-asana", this pose simply aids in releasing trapped gas in your digestive system.

Instructions:

- Lie flat on your back while relaxing at the same time.

- Bend your right knee slowly; use both your hands with interlocking fingers to bring it up towards your torso. Leave your left leg in its original position, flat on the floor.

- Your head and shoulders should be off the floor, while your chin must touch your right knee.

- Inhale slowly and hold it for few seconds then exhale as you return and lie flat on your back, while still holding your right knee.

- Rest for few seconds and repeat the same routine with your left leg.

4.   The Locust or Grasshopper Pose

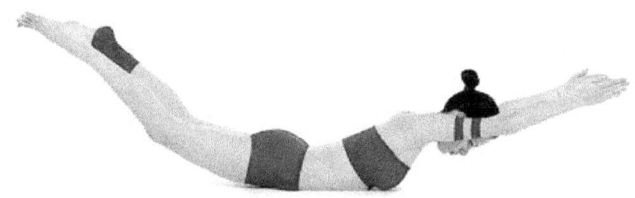

Photo Source: Wikimedia Commons

Its Sanskrit name is "Shalabha-asana" which represents a locust or a grasshopper.

Instructions:

- Lie flat on your stomach. Your head must be straight, and then tilt your forehead as you gently place your chin on your mat.

- Your arms are tucked sideways with palms facing upward. Gently slide your hands right beneath your thighs with your palms slowly pressing against your thighs. This is to support your legs later on when raising it. You can also bring your hands forward, as in the picture above.

- As you inhale slowly and deeply, try to raise altogether your head, chest and legs as high as you can off the floor while keeping your knees, thighs and feet all pressed together.

- Hold your breath while you maintain such position and slowly get back to your resting position while exhaling slowly.

5.   The Lion Pose

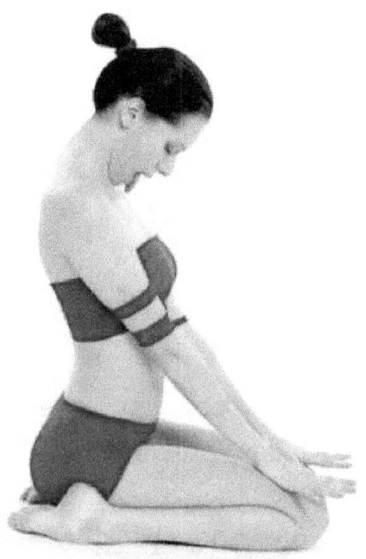

Photo Source: Wikimedia Commons

This pose represents the powerful one, which is the Lion. The Sanskrit name is "Simha-asana" which means a powerful being.

Instructions:

- Sit on your knees with your shins resting flat on the floor, and your buttocks gently pressed or resting against your heels.

- Place your hands on your knees while keeping a straight back, head and arms.

- Slowly lean forward while inhaling at the same time. Just like the Lion, stretch your jaws as wide as you can, stick your tongue out downward. Your gaze must be focused on the tip of your nose while stretching out only your fingers as far as you can from your knees.

- Hold such posture for a few seconds depending on how long you can hold your breath. Then exhale slowly while relaxing your body back to its original position.

6.   The Mountain Pose

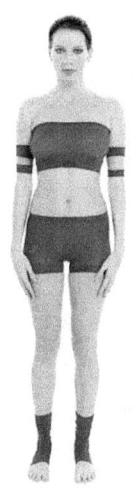

Photo Source: Wikimedia Commons

The level of difficulty is not as challenging as other postures; however this is perfect for beginners. It comes from the Sanskrit name "Tada-asana." In this pose you are expected to be standing firmly hence the name of The Mountain Pose.

Instructions:

- Stand erect and proper, with both feet flat on the floor. Your arms must be pressed on your sides while your palms are faced inward.

- Start flexing your thigh muscles as well as your stomach and the muscles in your buttocks. Your knees must also be flexed tightly to ensure a firm pose while balancing your weight effectively on both feet.

- As soon as you're ready, try to slowly lift your buttocks, arch your back gently while thrusting your abdominal muscles forward. Make sure to tilt back your head without losing balance.

7.   The Diamond Pose

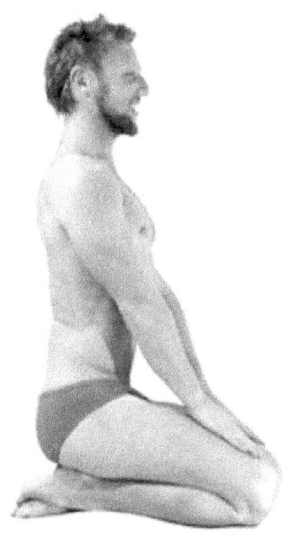

Photo Source: Wikimedia Commons

This pose is otherwise known in Sanskrit language as the "Vajra-asana." This means diamond as its English name suggests, or the thunderbolt.

Instructions:

- Bend your knees and sit on your heels. Make sure to place your knees apart, and the same goes for your legs and feet.

- With an erect back, place your hands right on your thighs with your palms face down.

- Breathe in and out comfortably in this relaxing position for as long as three minutes.

8. The Downward Dog Pose

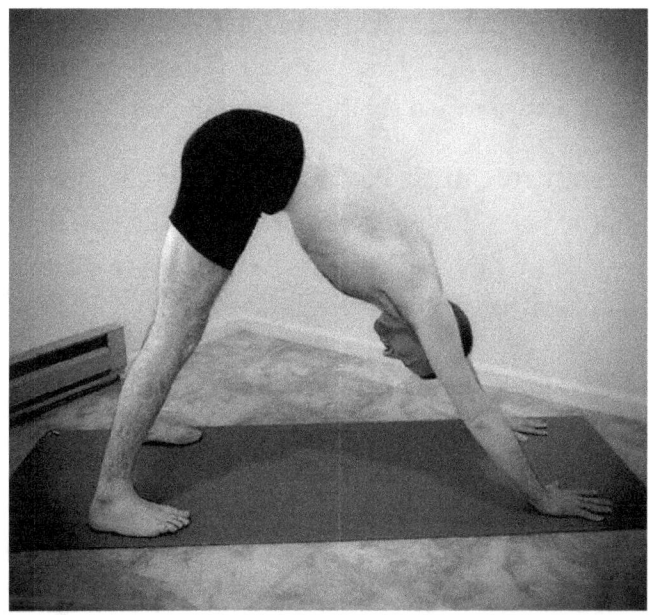

Photo Source: Wikimedia Commons

Its Sanskrit name is "Adho Mukha Svanasana." It focuses more on the balance of your arms as you bend forward.

Instructions:

- You need to position your body where your hands are situated under your shoulders and your knees below your hips.

- You must bend over and place your palms flat on your mat, with all your fingers widely separated. Move your hands forward for just a few inches.

- Your feet must be widely apart and your knees bent a little to observe an inverted letter V position. Move your thighs closer to your navel.

9. The Warrior I Pose

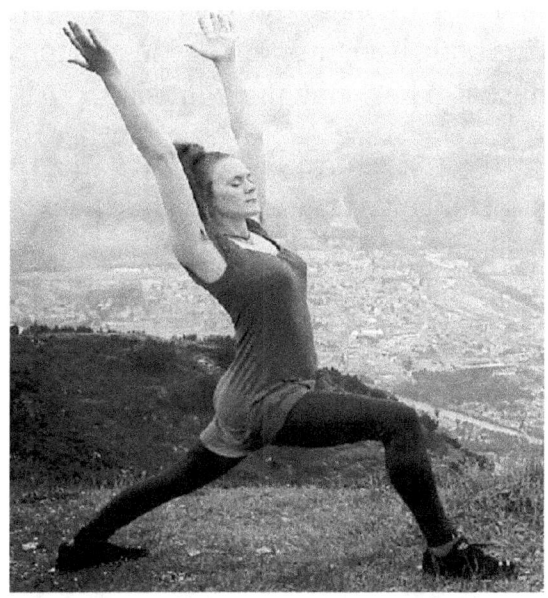

Photo Source: Wikimedia Commons

The Warrior Pose is comprised of three variations and it symbolizes the spiritual warrior within you. Its Sanskrit name is "Virabhadrasana I."

Instructions:

- Your feet must be placed apart at three to four feet distance.

- Your left foot must be positioned 60 degrees facing the right side, while your right foot must be 90 degrees facing the same direction as your left foot. Make sure both heels are aligned. Your torso must also be facing the right side.

- Your arms must be raised up, perpendicular to the floor while actively reaching out for the ceiling. Your head must stay in a neutral position.

- Stay in such position for a minute and repeat the same on your left side.

10. The Warrior II Pose

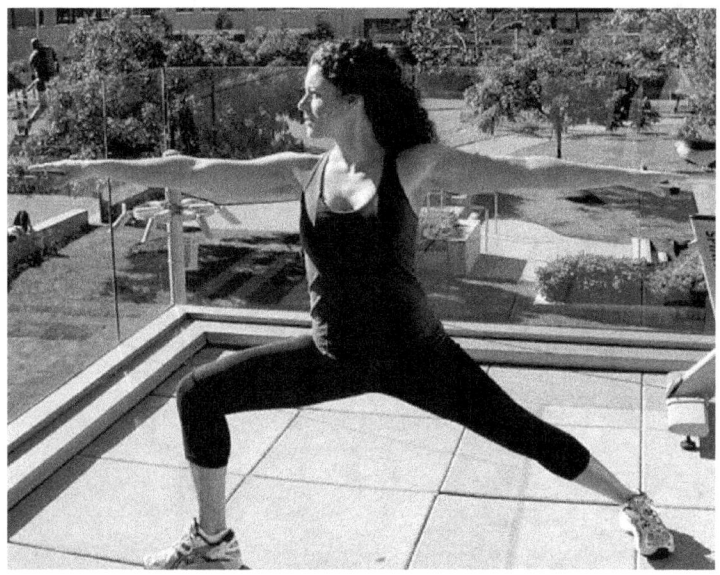

Photo Source: Wikimedia Commons

Just like its first variation, the Warrior II Pose has a Sanskrit name of "Virabhadrasana II." It is intended to strengthen your leg muscles, hips and even chest.

Instructions:

- Feet apart with about three to four feet distance. Place your right foot in an outward 90-degree position, while your left foot in a slightly inward position.

- Your hands and shoulders must equally be relaxed as you extend it out to your sides, with palms facing downward. Try to reach for the walls.

- Make sure your hips are sunk down towards the direction of the floor.

- Stay for a minute and switch sides slowly yet comfortably.

11.   The Tree Pose

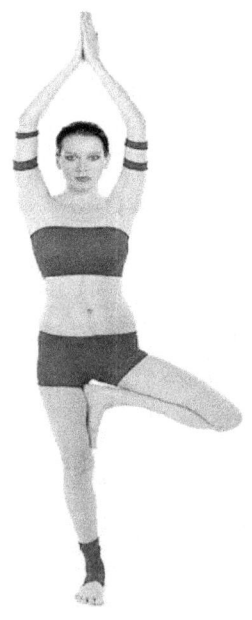

Photo Source: Wikimedia Commons

This posture comes from the Sanskrit name "Vriksha-asana." This is perfect for beginners, however some considers it as slightly tricky due to the required balancing ability when performing such pose.

Instructions:

- Start with your feet together while your arms placed at your sides.

- Bend your right knee and raise it slowly, bringing the right sole of your foot thigh high and inside position.

- Your left foot must balance your overall weight. Slowly raise your arms over your head. Make sure your elbows are not bent; make it as straight as possible until your palms are together above your head.

- Balance and hold your posture, you need to breathe in and out for at least 10 sets. Once done, pause and do the same routine on your opposite leg.

12.   The Wheel Pose

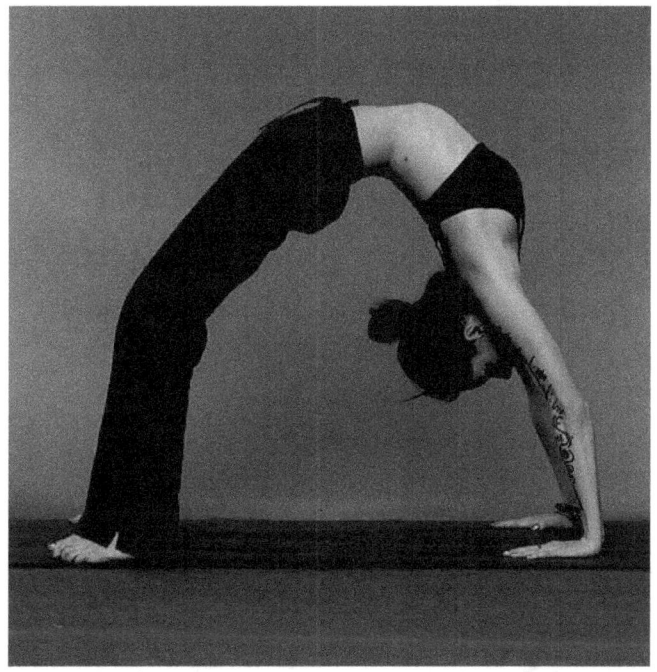

Photo Source: Wikimedia Commons

Although this is a challenging posture, many considers it as a must do for most beginners. When trying this out, it does not require you to successfully accomplish this pose, even if you fail to achieve this pose it still comes with amazing benefits. So beginners should not worry about trying this out. Just try your best.

Its Sanskrit name is "Chakra-asana" which means to move.

Instructions:

- Lie flat on your back. As you exhale, gently bend your knees and move your feet closer to your buttocks as you can. Make sure the soles of your feet are flat.

- Gently bend your elbows; the palms of your hand must be flat on the floor, which must be directly beneath your shoulders. Your fingers must also be directed towards the back.

- As you inhale deeply, slowly raise your head up along with your buttocks and back off the floor. Your spine should start to arch. Make use of your hands and feet to press in a downward direction to raise your stomach area and hips as high as you possibly can.

- If you find it uncomfortable to breathe in, slowly breathe out and return to your resting position of your back on the floor.

13. The Bridge Pose

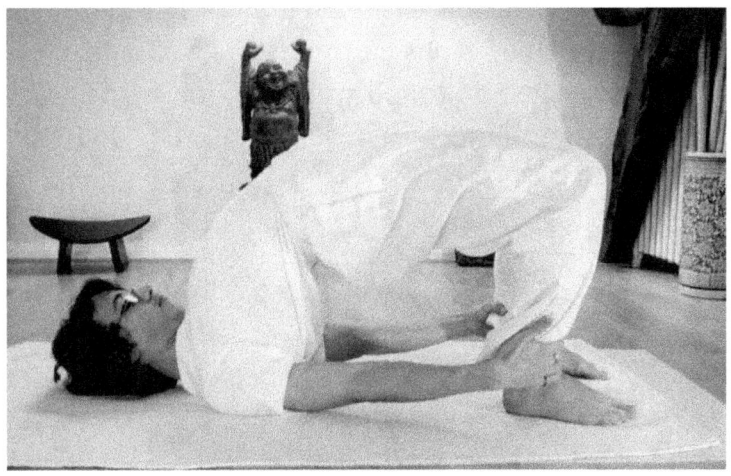

Photo Source: Wikimedia Commons

This is one of the gentle yoga poses for beginners that use gravity to expand the areas of your lungs and chest. Its Sanskrit name is "Setu Bandha Sarvangasana."

Instructions:

- As you lie on the floor, try to bend your knees.

- Your arms must be placed at your sides with each of your palms facing downward.

- Slowly press your feet and arms against the floor as you lift your hips upward, while exhaling at the same time.

- Make sure that your thighs are parallel to the floor. Your chin must be closer to your chest and hold your position for at least a minute.

14. The Seated Twist Pose

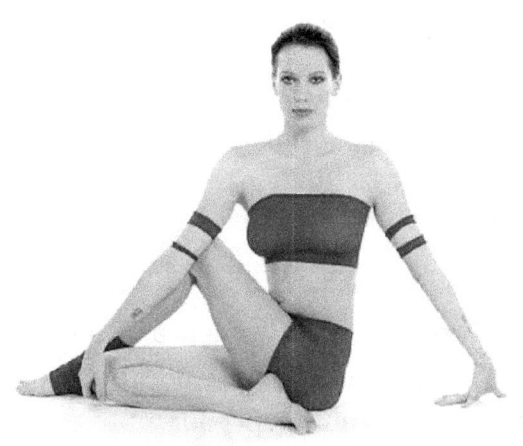

Photo Source: Wikimedia Commons

This pose is focused more on your shoulders. It also stretches your hips and back as well as enhancing blood circulation. Your abdomen is also given much attention as it tones it while strengthening your oblique muscles. This pose is known as "Ardha Matsyendrasana."

Instructions:

- As you sit on the floor, ensure that your legs are extended.

- Your right foot must cross over your left thigh with your left knee bent accordingly. Your right knee must point upward toward the ceiling.

- Your left elbow must then be placed outside your right knee, while your other hand securely touches the floor for balance just behind you.

- Now try to twist as much as you can, slowly feel the movement from your abdomen as you keep your butt firmly seated on the floor. This should last for a minute before switching sides.

15. The Cobra Pose

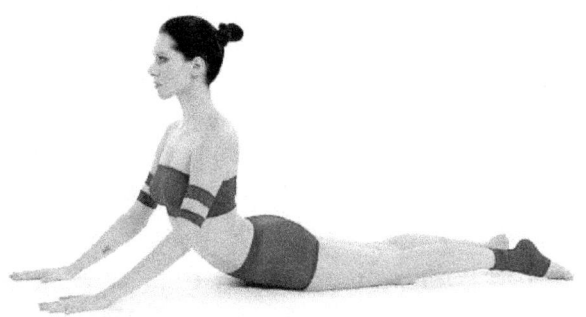

Photo Source: Wikimedia Commons

Doing this pose is great for your spine, chest and even lower back. This pose also stretches the chest muscles. This pose has the Sanskrit name of "Naga-asana."

Instructions:

- Comfortably lie on your stomach. Your head must be turned to one side while your arms are positioned alongside your body. Your thumbs must be positioned right under your shoulders. Extend your legs gently ensuring that the top of your feet lie flat on the floor.

- Gently squeeze your gluteus muscles; your hips must be tucked downward as you continue to strengthen your pelvic area.

- Firmly press your shoulders down and push your hands strongly to raise your chest upward, raising your torso starting from your waist area off the floor. Your spine must arch backwards slowly and you eventually straighten your arms while your hips are still touching on the floor.

- Be calm, relax and repeat the same routine as needed.

16. The Crow Position

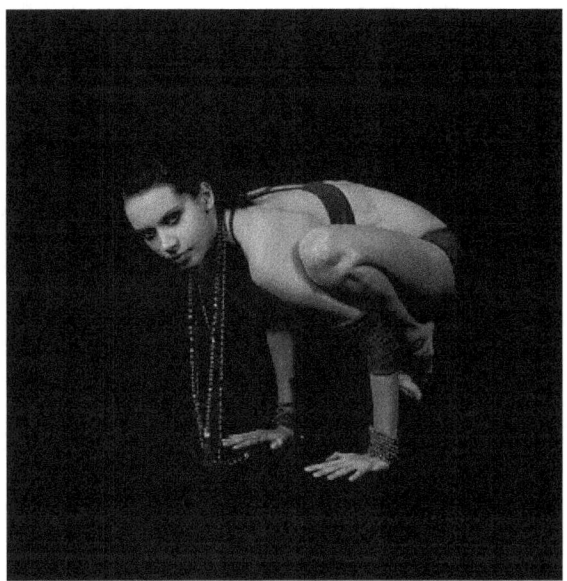

Photo Source: Wikimedia Commons

This pose comes with an intermediate level of difficulty; beginners can still work on this pose. It focuses more on your arm balance, which also involves your shoulders and core. Its Sanskrit name is "Bakasana" which means crane.

Instructions:

- Position into the downward dog pose where your palms and feet are pressed firmly on the floor.

- Once balance is gained, slowly walk your feet towards your arms until your knees touch it.

- Your elbows must be bent slowly, at the same time your heels lifted off from the floor. Abdomen is engaged while your legs are strongly pressed adjacent to your arms.

- Hold such position until you have completed 5 to 10 breaths

17. The Pigeon Pose

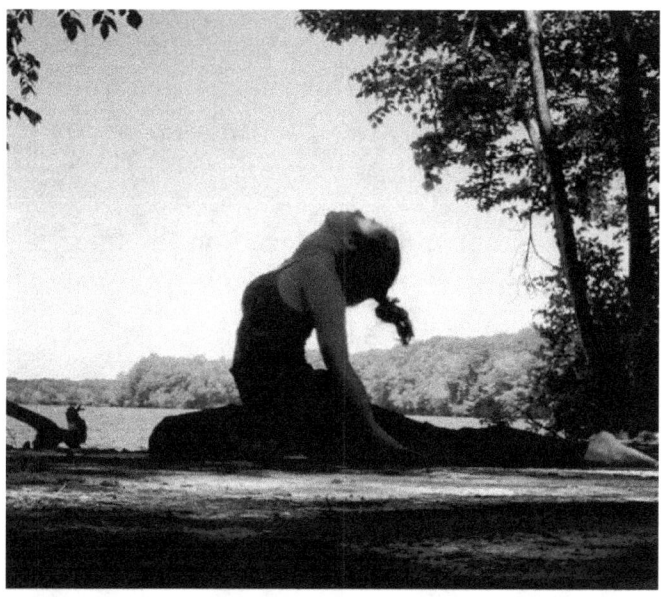

Photo Source: Wikimedia Commons

Just like the Cobra Pose, this one also focuses on your shoulder strength. It helps stretch your chest muscles and perfect for quad stretch too. Its Sanskrit name is "Eka pada rajakapotasana."

Instructions:

- Position yourself in a push up pose. Your palms must be placed under your shoulders.

- Your right heel must be positioned right on your left hip. This means that your left knee should be on the floor extended.

- Your hands must be placed on the floor, pressing gently as you raise or lift your chest while sitting back.

18. The Half Moon Pose

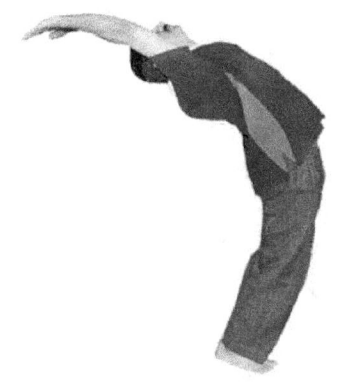

Photo Source: Wikimedia Commons

This pose focuses on basic balancing, while also stretching muscles in the chest and abdomen. Its Sanskrit name is "Ardhachundra-asana."

Instructions:

- Stand erect with your toes and heels flat on the floor.

- Your back should be straight and your arms placed on your sides with inward facing palms.

- Slowly bring your hands right on your chest, see to it that your palms are against each other and slightly pressed.

- As you inhale, raise both hands without bending them while arching your back while your arms are slowly positioning alongside your neck and head.

- Don't forget to tilt your head slightly backward and hold your position as you keep your knees firmly straight. Then go back to your resting position slowly.

19.   The King of the Dance Pose

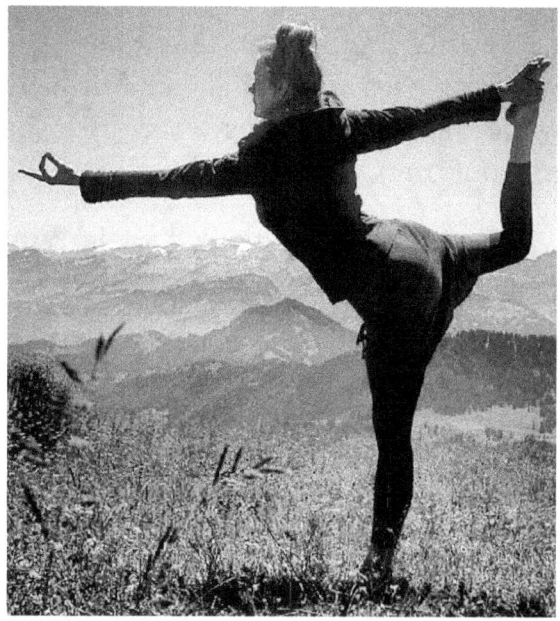

Photo Source: Wikimedia Commons

This pose is quite fun, you can perform it as if you are dancing gracefully. Your spine will receive all the benefits as it aligns your vertebrae and eases strain felt due to poor body posture caused by prolonged periods of sitting. Its Sanskrit name is "Nataraja-asana."

Instructions:

- Stand straight with your feet together and your arms placed at your sides.

- Slowly bend your right leg in a backwards motion; at the same time reach your left foot using your left hand while slowly extending your opposite arm out front.

- Make sure your extended right arm reaches a 90 degrees angle from the floor as you lift your left leg as high as you can while using your left arm.

- Steady your position as you breathe in and out using your nostrils. You can do this for a minute and slowly return to your standing position.

20. The Corpse Pose

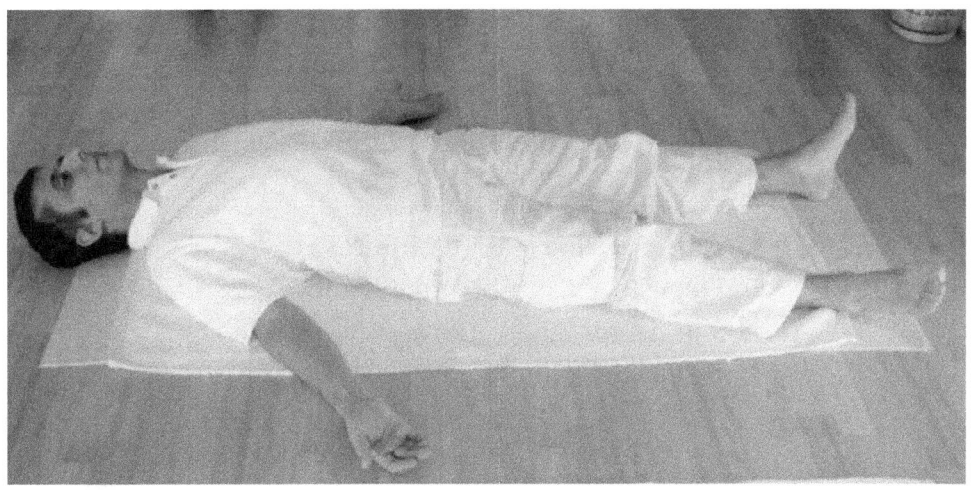

Photo Source: Wikimedia Commons

The goal of this pose is to achieve a perfectly relaxed mind and still body. Your body needs to be motionless and your mind as quiet as possible. Its Sanskrit name is "Shava-asana."

Instructions:

- You need to lie on your back as flat as you can with your legs placed together, but not touching each other. Your arms must be out to your side or close to your body and your palms must be facing up.

- Close your eyes, achieve relaxed facial muscles as you continue to breathe in and out with your nostrils, slowly and comfortably.

- With conscious effort, bring your full attention to every part of your body starting from your head.

- Remain still for 3 to 5 minutes. In case you feel sleepy, simply inhale and exhale faster than normal to awaken your senses again.

Conclusion

Yoga does not really require you to use any equipment. Instead it makes you get in touch with your inner strength. Make use of your body to discover your capacity, push your limits and transform from within. If you want real transformation, yoga is your best option. You can simply do it indoors, at home, inside a studio, or in the office. You can also do it outdoors to make it more fun and to connect effectively with your body as well as nature. After familiarizing yourself with the basic yoga postures provided, you will be feeling much better psychically, mentally and emotionally. Remember to take your time and hold positions for as long as you feel comfortable.

I hope this book was able to impact your life in a positive way. The next step is to keep practicing and you will see results!

Finally, if you enjoyed this book, then I'd like to ask you for a favor. Would you be kind enough to leave a review for this book on Amazon? It really helps me out and is greatly appreciated!

Thank you and good luck!

Here Are My Other Best Selling Books On Amazon!

Below you'll find some of my other best selling books on Amazon and Kindle as well.

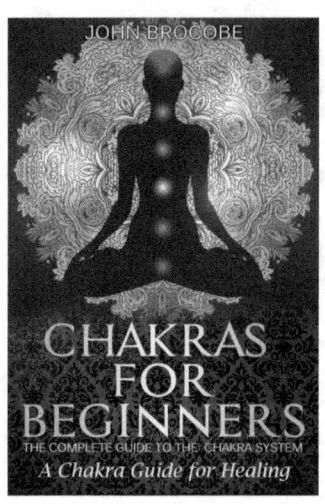

Chakras for Beginners: The Complete Guide to the Chakra System

Go to: amzn.to/1SIvGpu

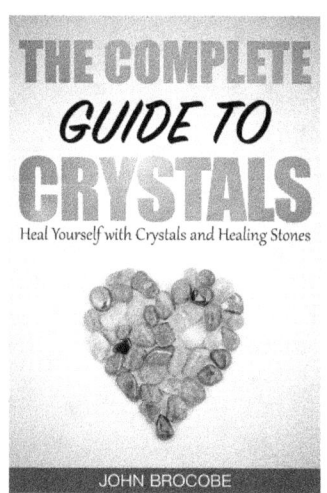

Crystals: The Complete Guide to Crystals: Heal Yourself with Crystals and Healing Stones

Go to: amzn.to/1JzHpoJ

www.ingramcontent.com/pod-product-compliance
Lightning Source LLC
Chambersburg PA
CBHW071248280526
45788CB00004B/1625